Ali Kicking

Andy Legg

ACCENT PRESS LTD

Introduction

They say that one in three people will suffer from cancer. The trouble is, you never believe you will be the one. I certainly didn't. Why should I?

When I was first diagnosed with cancer I had been a professional footballer for more than ten years. I wasn't the most skilful player you will ever see, but I always gave 100 per cent and took pride in my fitness.

Some footballers have to be really careful about what they eat to ensure they don't put on the pounds. But I never had to worry about that – burgers or pies never seemed to touch me. I was naturally fit and athletic, almost without having to try.

And I was blessed with a valuable added weapon for football – a long throw – which earned me a place in the *Guinness Book of Records*. It was a gift which, in my opinion, was another sign of my fitness.

All this helped me enjoy my football career. I went late into the game, having had 'proper jobs' before being taken on as a professional by Swansea City. Because I had seen working life outside the game, I think I appreciated the life of a footballer more than some of those who had turned professional immediately after they had left school.

It was a wonderful life. I loved playing football for a living and I loved the training, too. Whether it was boiling hot or freezing cold, I was in the fresh air kicking a ball around.

Frankly, I didn't have a care in the world. I made a lot of friends in the game, joined some terrific clubs and, though I was never fortunate enough to play in the Premier League, I was well paid for playing a game I enjoyed. I was also proud that I had played for my country.

With a wonderful family to go with a comfortable living I felt very fortunate. Other than the usual football injuries I didn't worry about my health. I was a footballer who could run around as energetically as any of the youngsters who were just coming into the game.

So cancer was the very last thing on my mind. It was something which affected others. It is hard to believe now, but even when my first neck tumour appeared in the winter of

1999, I didn't give it a second thought.

The lump wasn't painful, it didn't affect my ability to do my job, and unless you looked closely you couldn't see it. I just ignored it and it was only because I was nagged so much that I had it looked at and then taken away.

In truth even that didn't bother me. I was still playing in the Football League, was still fit and once it had gone I put it out of my mind.

Yet cancer was to return just a few years later. In this book, I have spoken as plainly as I can about my fight against cancer. Some of the detail is still painful for me to recall.

I have not written this either to frighten people or for sympathy. I have gone into detail partly to pay tribute to the medical experts who saved my life and who continue to save more lives today.

I am here because of their work and dedication. And they are still helping me to fight cancer because they and I know that it could return at any time. And there are many others like me. I am sure their outlook on life has changed, just like mine. I'm still positive. I'm still fighting and I am trying to do as much as I can to help other people overcome the condition.

I hope while reading this book you will get my message of hope. I have always felt lucky about my life and still do now. My family are fantastic, my career has been in a game little boys dream about playing – and I have survived a disease some people don't even like mentioning.

I am living proof that cancer does not have to be a death sentence. If it can be caught early enough it can be dealt with, such is the improvement in medical care over the last few years. My cancer fight has shown me just how much the experts can do and how much people care.

When I was at my lowest, I received a great deal of support, particularly from football fans. Some of these same fans would hurl abuse at me when I was playing against their team. But that was just football. When I was ill their messages of support were uplifting to me and helped keep me going.

This may surprise some, but I know, from personal experience, football supporters don't always deserve the reputation they've been given in some quarters. So this book is also a 'thank you' to all the fans who took the time to send me, a person who they had only seen playing football, their best wishes when they became aware of my illness. Their response continues to be an inspiration to me.

The fans, the continued care of the experts and the support of my family and friends are the reasons why I am 'Alive and Kicking' today.

Chapter One

The Initial Shock

It was my wife Lucy who first saw the lump. One morning I was in the bathroom shaving. "You've got a lump on your neck," she said. I couldn't feel a thing.

But she insisted that when I lifted my chin to shave in the corners, she could see a lump. "You need to go and get that checked out. Go and see the doctor about it." However, the words went in one ear and out the other.

I was blasé about it. It was the Christmas of 1999 and I was playing for Cardiff City, thoroughly enjoying my football at a club where, after initial hostility from the fans, I had now settled.

As a professional footballer I knew one of my assets was high energy and fitness. I didn't feel at all ill. I didn't give a little lump on my neck any thought, particularly as it didn't give me any pain. Seems ridiculous to say this now, but I didn't worry about such things.

Lucy was pregnant at the time and I was more concerned about her. But she was determined I should get it looked at and she even tried to embarrass me by getting her midwife to add her voice and push me to get it seen. I ignored them both. Nobody else noticed the lump and I just got on with my life. In fact I was sure the lump was all to do with a wisdom tooth which had broken through.

Lucy has much more sense than me. If she sees anything wrong she wants it sorted out, whereas I have always had a 'couldn't care less' outlook on life.

I didn't even think about cancer. I had never come across the disease – there was no history of anything like that in my family.

Looking back, I suppose I was just naïve, though the fact that I didn't worry meant I always had a positive attitude, and they reckon that always helps when facing illness.

But, of course, I didn't consider anything was actually wrong. It was the wisdom tooth, nothing more.

Lucy didn't give up. And she insisted, "It's getting bigger." She was probably right, but still I couldn't feel anything. It wasn't affecting my form on the pitch so I dismissed all thoughts of it, until one midweek evening game at Ninian Park.

I went into the medical room to have some strapping put on, as footballers do before a match, and the club doctor Len Noakes was there with another doctor. Len asked him to look at the lump and he said I should see someone about it.

Len organised for me to go to the BUPA Hospital in Cardiff and see a specialist called Alan Jones. He wanted me to have a biopsy to check what the lump actually was.

I will always remember the day I went to the hospital because Lucy rang me as I was getting out of the car. "Are you there?" she asked. I told her I was, but I'm not sure she believed me. She wanted proof. I had to find a nurse and get her to talk to my wife on the phone to confirm I had actually gone to the hospital – and wasn't somewhere else playing a game of golf!

Lucy knew how much I hated hospitals and needles in particular. As a footballer I like to think I never shirked a tackle, took the bumps and bruises as part of the game, and always enjoyed the physical side of the sport, even if sometimes it meant getting hurt.

But hospitals? No, thank you.

But here I was, and once I'd convinced my wife I was actually going ahead with the biopsy, I went in and had the lump looked at.

The results came back a few days later. I was told it was a non-malignant tumour and I was pleased to hear the doctor wasn't worried about it since by this time we were coming close to the end of the season. We agreed I should finish the campaign at Cardiff and then have an operation to have the lump taken away.

I can't remember whether the word 'cancer' was mentioned. And I'm not even sure I told Lucy it could be cancerous. That's how laid back about it I was.

The only thing which worried me was having to go into hospital to have the lump taken out, because I knew that would involve needles and other medical stuff. So I put it all to the back of my mind and continued my football at Cardiff, finishing the season and then getting ready to have the lump dealt with.

In that season the club were fighting relegation so I was concentrating on that, plus my wife's pregnancy. The only people at Cardiff who were aware of the tumour were Len Noakes, the club physio Mike Davenport and the manager Billy Ayre. They all agreed to keep quiet about it and not tell the other players. The lump would be removed and then I would tell people the whole story.

For the operation, I went to the BUPA Hospital in Cardiff, but when I checked in they told me I was actually having the surgery at the Princess of Wales Hospital in Bridgend. So going private was a bit of a waste of time for me.

At the Princess of Wales I was put in a ward with other patients and I was quite pleased with that. I know some people like private rooms in hospital, but I didn't want to be on my own.

I was in overnight, had the operation and Lucy came to pick me up. When she asked how it had gone, there was the usual blank from me. I told her there was nothing to worry about, it had all been taken away and I certainly wasn't going to be bothered by it. My only concern was the warning from the surgeon that because they had had to cut nerves in the neck I might lose some feeling on the right-hand side of my face. Other than that, and the fact that it was a bit sore, I was unconcerned.

Now, I realise how much of a worry I must have been to those who were close to me. I get annoyed with myself about just how stupid I was. There I was, facing what was potentially a life-threatening illness and I just did not consider what the consequences might have been for my wife or my family. I shudder to think what might have happened had I ignored the lump altogether.

But, after having the operation in May 2000, I got the all clear from the doctor. He was pleased with the way the operation had gone and, though the tumour had been cancerous, it was confirmed as benign. Since the doctor was happy, I was, too.

The only sign of the operation was a scar on my neck which was pretty long, but that was to be expected in a soft tissue area. Straight after the surgery I had to be careful with my head and neck, but that discomfort didn't last long.

With the operation out of the way I had other things on my mind. My daughter Alicia had been born in March and I was enjoying looking after her.

And as far as the football was concerned, I was bang on schedule to be back in time for pre-season training. I was raring to go for the new season with Cardiff City.

Chapter Two

More Bad News

It was about four years later, when I had left Cardiff City and my family and I had gone to live in Nottingham, that I realised something might be wrong again.

I was playing for Peterborough at the time. I mentioned to my wife that I could feel another little lump developing in the same place where I had had the original operation.

Of course Lucy wanted me to get it examined immediately. I told her to wait and see – so we left it. And the lump got bigger. This time even I realised that.

Because Len Noakes, the doctor at Cardiff, knew my history, I decided to contact him. He told me it was pointless coming back to Cardiff to have it looked at, and said he would recommend someone nearer to my home. Luckily, Len had done his homework and, as I was later to discover, I ended up seeing one of the top head and neck cancer specialists in Britain.

Patrick Bradley was an Irishman who was based at the Nuffield Hospital in Nottingham. He was an absolutely great guy with a terrific personality who was up front and positive, and I got on with him straight away. He also treated the cricketer Geoffrey Boycott when he had cancer and was definitely one of the top people in his field.

On my first visit to Patrick he had a look at the lump and didn't think there was too much to worry about. He advised me to have a biopsy but, just as at Cardiff a few years earlier, I was keen to see out the season with my club Peterborough. I told the manager Barry Fry I would play on and get it looked at during the close season.

But things took a turn for the worse in January 2005, when I was playing against Oldham at Peterborough's London Road ground. I actually scored in the match but later, when I jumped up for a ball, I got caught by a stray elbow in the throat and it hit me right on the lump.

I winced because, for the first time, it hurt me. I'd never felt pain there before and thought, "That didn't feel good." In fact it hurt me so much I remember kicking the player afterwards. I smashed him because he'd caused me pain and the referee showed me a red card!

I continued to play, but the lump now started to feel sore and every time I took a knock on that part of my neck it hurt. So I went to see Patrick Bradley and told him about it. He wanted me to come in right away to get the lump taken out.

Barry Fry told me to book myself in for surgery immediately. I remember doing it as I travelled for a game to Hartlepool, which turned out to be my second-from-last match as a Football League player.

On 9 April 2005 I played in Peterborough's 1–0 win at Blackpool and, though I didn't know it at the time, this was my last game as a professional footballer. A few days later I had the operation at the Queen's Medical Centre in Nottingham.

They told me they could get me seen quicker under the National Health Service, so once again going private had been a waste of time.

I've already mentioned about my fear of needles and hospitals. When I went in for the surgery I can remember, just as the anaesthetist was about to put the needle in, the doctor said to me, "You know when we cut your scar again you may lose some of the feeling from your nerves in your face and neck." As he said that, I was injected and knocked out. He knew I wouldn't have gone through with it had I known it earlier.

I remember waking up and feeling horrible, as you do after operations, I suppose. I didn't feel particularly sore, but I did feel numbness. In fact I couldn't feel any part of that side of my face or neck and that was a worry. I wondered when feeling would return.

The next day the doctor came to see me, took the drip out and sent me home. But within a few hours one side of my face filled up like a balloon. I looked like the Elephant Man. There was a build-up of fluid because I was still bleeding internally.

Lucy rushed me back into hospital and, as if things weren't already bad enough, they made me swallow a little camera. It was horrible and I had to be goaded into it, the nurse giving me stick, calling me a 'poof' because I was scared, and Lucy saying I was acting like a baby. Didn't they realise what I was going through?

Throughout my career as a footballer, I'd only suffered two broken legs. I'd been to hospital to have plasters put on and that was it. Now I was really suffering, even though I knew they had to deal with the problem. They were worried the build-up of blood might block my airways.

They kept me in another night and when everything had calmed down and my face looked a little more like it had before the surgery, I was sent home and had to wait for the results.

I suppose I had a sense things could be more serious this time when I saw Patrick Bradley before leaving the hospital. He told me he wasn't entirely happy with the operation, because he had had to take out a lot more than he thought he would have to.

What he meant was that he had removed my lymph gland and saliva gland. His exact words were, "I've gone so deep I couldn't go any deeper."

What really worried me was an expression he used afterwards to sum up the whole scene inside my neck. "It looked lively," he said. To me that didn't sound good. The word "lively" really concerned me and for the first time I sensed I might not be as lucky as I had been last time.

So I was fearful, but couldn't let it show. I

kept my feelings to myself and didn't even tell Lucy of my private concerns. Then I had to endure the wait for the results of the examination of the lump which had been taken out.

Lucy and I went to see Patrick for the results a couple of days later. The wait had been difficult. When we got to the hospital, we actually saw him in the corridor and he said, "I'm glad you're here, I need to see you – go straight into my office." I'm sure my chin must have dropped, because I immediately sensed from Patrick's manner that I was about to receive bad news.

We did as we were told. Patrick walked in and, typical of the way he is, came straight out with it. "There's no kind way of telling you this ... you've got cancer."

I was numb. I just sat there. Lucy was silent, absolutely silent. The first lump a few years before had been removed and I had had no concerns. I hadn't felt as though I had cancer in my body because that tumour had been benign. This was very much a life-changing moment and I knew it.

After the initial shock, Patrick started to explain further. "I've cut out as much as I can, but you never know whether it will turn up somewhere else."

I was told I'd have to have a full body scan to check it wasn't elsewhere in my body. Because of his approach outside the office I'd almost prepared myself for what I had heard and I think I was lucky to have someone who came straight out with the truth. Patrick was blunt and I appreciated that, even though what I had heard was shocking.

Apparently the sort of cancer I had was rarely found, and even rarer in the lymph gland. It usually lived on nerve ends.

"What's the worst thing that could happen?" I asked him. He pulled no punches with his reply. "The worst thing is that it could be somewhere else." If that happened, Patrick said, the severity would depend on where it was.

"Above the jaw line or below the collar bone ... you're looking at possibly twelve to eighteen months," he said. He meant twelve to eighteen months to live. I told you he was blunt. But he was positive, too. Caught early enough, I would have years to live and he was happy the operation had gone well even though he had removed more than he had expected.

There are some days in your life you never forget. This was one of them. I somehow had to deal with the fact that I might have just eighteen months to live if things were really bad. It kept going over and over in my mind: "I might only have eighteen months to live."

I jumped in the car for the journey home and it really hit me. I'm not ashamed to say I had tears running down my face. I kept looking away from Lucy, who was driving. I was trying to hide my emotions. "There's no need to," she said. "It's a frightening thing."

That short trip home was the toughest journey of my life. I looked at the baby seat in the back of the car and it struck me I might never see my daughter grow up. My wife was obviously crying, too. We gave each other a hug and I said, "Let's hope for the best ... see if we can get through it."

Truthfully, that was me being more positive than I was feeling. I was hurting terribly inside. But I was glad we had the journey home together to try and get our minds around what had been said.

For the next few days I was in a bad way. Lucy kept asking me if I felt okay. But I just wanted to spend time by myself. I would make excuses to be alone, sit there staring into space and then build up enough courage to be positive again when I was with Lucy and Alicia.

I had cancer. The 'Big C' – an illness few people are comfortable talking about. I had to face up to that fact and I also had to brace myself for potentially more bad news.

Had all the cancer been removed from my neck? And was it elsewhere? Would my life be measured in years, or months?

Chapter Three

Cancer Treatment

I made another visit to the Nuffield Hospital, this time for the crucial examination.

I had to go for a full body scan to check whether the cancer was still present anywhere in my body. They were thorough, they had to be. I was totally enclosed in what they call an MRI tunnel for an hour and a half. It was one of the most stressful ninety minutes of my life.

I'm not good in hospitals and I really do not like having my movement restricted and being enclosed. I had to concentrate on keeping still, because if I moved or wriggled I might have to do it all again. Those who know me will realise how hard it is for me to keep still.

But it was worse waiting for the scan results. That was mental cruelty. All sorts of things go through your mind. I didn't know how ill or how close to death I might be.

We tried to keep everything hush-hush. I'd

told my immediate family, but kept the details to a close few. Of my friends, I think I only told fellow player Jason Bowen about the scans and what they might reveal.

Patrick Bradley was abroad at a conference when I was due to have the results. He rang me from there to check I'd received them, but I hadn't. As soon as he touched down back in Britain he rang to say he'd get straight in his car, get the results, and would ring me. My case was on his mind the moment he returned home, which for a busy man was unbelievable.

The phone rang and I'll never forget what he said. "I've had the results ... they look okay ... go and have a beer." Normally so positive, I turned all negative. I asked him what "okay" actually meant. He kept repeating his words. "They look okay ... go and have a beer."

I took his words to mean I was virtually clear, though he explained I still had to have a course of radiotherapy. Patrick's thoughts were to blast the area that had had the cancer to remove any remaining trace. Sounds simple, doesn't it? Little did I know what lay ahead.

Because the radiotherapy treatment can be so severe, they have to be spot-on, targeting the area they want to treat. And because of where my tumour was, I had to wear a face mask to protect me from the rays to stop them damaging other, healthy parts, of my face and neck. Radiotherapy kills everything and I certainly didn't want it killing things it shouldn't.

The mask was frightening in itself, because it was so tight to my skin. There was a little gap in it for them to insert a tube through which I could breathe. I've still got the mask now, a sort of keepsake to remind me how lucky I've been. And the discomfort didn't end there. I also had to wear a brace under my neck to keep my chin up. A picture I was not!

All this was bad enough. What they didn't tell me as we practised getting used to the mask was that they also had to bolt me to the bed for the treatment. I could hear the bolts turning and I was not impressed. I spat out the breathing tube and swore and shouted, "Get me out of here, I can't have that!"

They explained that if I moved, the radiotherapy might miss what it was supposed to hit and cause me even more damage. They had so much patience with me at the City Hospital in Nottingham. I can't really thank them enough – I don't think I was what you would call a model patient!

It took two or three weeks of preparation

before I actually started my treatment. During this time I wasn't allowed to wet shave with a razor. I had to dry shave because the treatment would thin the skin and that might cause problems.

After all the build-up and getting used to that mask, mentally I felt I was ready for everything.

The medical staff had warned me about the side effects of the radiotherapy treatment. Within the first week I might lose my sense of taste and my mouth would be dry. In the second week I would find it hard to swallow and in the weeks after that my throat would be red raw and I'd find it difficult to drink anything.

At the time I'd just knocked down my house and we were living in a static caravan in Nottingham, so it was a difficult time anyway. Now I had all of this to contend with.

I was due to have twenty-five treatments, five sessions a week, each one usually lasting just under twenty minutes.

After the first week I was feeling fine. I met other patients there who said they couldn't swallow and I was glad it wasn't affecting me as much as it appeared to affect them.

In the second week, however, I had a

strange taste of copper in my mouth and it was difficult to swallow because of the soreness in my throat. Week three and I could hardly eat. My wife was having to turn my food into liquid and was making me 'shakes' to drink.

By week four I couldn't believe how hard it was. I was in too much pain to swallow food and I wasn't even able to drink water. Unless you have been through this, it is difficult to understand how you can be in agony even swallowing your own saliva. But that is the way it was. The pain was awful and there was no escape from it.

Though the radiotherapy sessions were just a few minutes each day, the pain wore me down and I constantly felt tired. Sometimes I would go back to the caravan and just not move. Only a few months previously I had been running around football pitches and being put through my paces nearly every day in training. Now all I wanted to do was lie down. And all the time there was this burning sensation in my throat. I'd never experienced anything like it.

So the last thing I wanted to hear after reaching twenty treatments was that they wanted to increase the number to thirty-two!

I didn't think I could cope. I didn't have

much weight to lose anyway, but the pounds were dropping off me and my mood had changed. From being happy-go-lucky, the nurses now thought I was Mr Grumpy.

"Here comes the miserable git," they'd say, just to try to make me laugh and raise my spirits. They know what people go through with this treatment.

It was the toughest time of my life and one morning I'd just had enough. I told them the treatment that day would definitely be my last. I needed to eat but couldn't because of the pain and it was getting too much to bear.

They told me to take a couple of days off from treatment and even offered to give me a food bag to attach to my stomach so I could be fed that way. "No chance," I said. Sounds stupid and pig-headed now because I was in pain and loads of people have these bags. But it was something I didn't even want to think about.

I started feeling sorry for myself.

I started to wonder why someone who had never smoked and who had been fit and healthy had been hit by cancer. It didn't seem fair. I was angry and couldn't understand why it had happened to me.

But then my radiotherapy session was

changed from the usual morning to the afternoon – they told me the machine was being serviced. I was at my lowest, until I walked into hospital for my treatment. There I saw a young girl who could have been no more than six or seven years old. She was obviously having radiotherapy and chemotherapy, and she'd lost all her hair. Yet she was smiling and looking happy.

I suddenly thought to myself, Why am I moaning? Even if I "pop my clogs" soon I've had a great life. All I had to worry about was my wife and daughter. Compared to the life I had enjoyed, that little girl had had nothing, yet was smiling as she went through hell. I stopped feeling sorry for myself the minute I saw her. Yes, I was still moody, but she gave me a different outlook.

To this day I don't know whether the nurses planned it and I don't know who the girl was or what happened to her. But I've always been sure the nurses had something to do with me being there while she was there, and the minute I saw her it hit home that whatever problems I had, there's always someone who is worse off.

However, after twenty-eight treatments I threw in the towel. Lucy told me to think about my family and to think again, but I'd reached the point of no return. The doctor tried to talk me out of it but I was adamant, I could not go on. The next day I took in some chocolates and thanked the nurses for all they had done for me. I went back to Patrick Bradley who said, "I can't believe you didn't get to thirty-two sessions." I told him I was a bit ashamed myself. But then he and the other doctor smiled and told me I'd done well to get to twenty-eight with little food and no food bag. I'd endured more than they thought I would. The most difficult period of my life was over. I'd gone through turmoil, physically and mentally. With the medical help I'd managed to get through it.

I was peeved about one thing – I had had to quit full-time professional football. That upset me because it was not my choice. I had been forced out of my livelihood through no fault of my own. It wasn't as if I had had to pack in because of a football injury, which does happen in the sport. My case was different.

I had told Peterborough boss Barry Fry as soon as they'd found the cancer that I wouldn't be able to go on. I just wouldn't have the fitness needed to continue playing at that level.

But, thinking about it now, having to drop

out of the Football League was a small price to pay. Thanks to people like Patrick Bradley and the other medical staff who dealt with me, I was still alive – if not kicking!

Chapter Four

Support from the Football "Family"

It was an eye-opener to see the work of the medical teams with cancer patients. Their patience, understanding, will and dedication is truly amazing.

But there is more to dealing with the illness than just coping with the treatment physically. You need mental strength, too. I was grateful for the support of my close friends and family, which was unstinting. But I also had help from the football world.

Football fans often have a bad press and attract unwanted headlines. But I experienced another side to them. I have nothing but praise for those football followers who took time out to send me messages of support when I was fighting my second tumour and coping with the treatment which followed.

When I told the Peterborough manager Barry Fry I had cancer, he immediately released it to the media and I had loads of calls. The staff at Cardiff City were soon on the phone to me, as were people from some of my other former clubs.

Frank Burrows, who managed me at Swansea and Cardiff, lifted my spirits when he sent a card wishing me well. He left the price tag on it and just under the marker for £1.68 he added, "This card cost me more than what I paid you at Swansea!" And he wasn't far wrong. Bobby Gould, in charge of me at Cardiff and Wales, was also quick to get in touch and stayed in contact throughout.

When news of my illness broke in the media, there were pages and pages of 'get well' messages in the Cardiff-based *South Wales Echo*. I sort of expected them from Cardiff City fans, because by the end of my time at Ninian Park they were great with me. But what shocked me was the rest of the football supporters who sent me messages of support.

I had many from Bristol City fans, which staggered me. I had always been a target for the boo-boys whenever I played against them. Remember, I had been part of the Cardiff team which had beaten them in the play-off semi-final – our win completed at Ashton Gate. Yet, here I was, feeling terrible and having my spirits lifted by messages of goodwill from supporters who had been angry with me and the rest of the Cardiff players that night, and on other occasions.

They weren't just wishing me well, they would frequently add messages which were positive and encouraging. One said, "We always hated you, but we wanted you on our team because you're a fighter." Another said, "You used to kick people – you can kick this too."

Typical was an anonymous 'get well' card which said, "I had never heard of you until yesterday when I read the newspaper. I looked at your reports on the internet and you were a fighter on the pitch – I am sure you can beat this." It was signed 'An Arsenal Fan'.

I had messages from supporters connected to all the clubs I played for, such as those based in the 'Jimmy Sirrell Stand' at Notts County, but also many from others I had never been associated with. Most surprising for me were those I had from football supporters around the world – as far afield as New Zealand, Australia and America.

The fans who contacted me will never realise how much those messages of support meant, and how much they helped me in my time of real need. Whenever I was feeling under the weather, which was often during my radiotherapy, Lucy and I would get out the cards and e-mails and read through them. They were an inspiration to us both as we battled through that difficult time.

It goes to show that the tribal rivalry in football means nothing when things are really serious. Fans hammer different players every week. You are a target, you are there to be shot at simply by pulling on a football shirt and playing in front of a crowd who have paid money to watch you.

Some fans used to show their hostility towards me to try to put me off, so I wouldn't play well against them. But, as some of the messages said, that was showing me a kind of respect.

When I was struck by cancer, my plight was known because I was a footballer. I would never have had all those e-mails, cards and messages if I hadn't played the game at a reasonable level, which led to the media interest. But my health problems were above and beyond football, they were far more important. And when I most needed them, those same people who had given me flak and directed their abuse at me from the terraces were there to support me.

I hope that those who did take the time in their busy lives to send those messages will accept my public thanks for their support.

Of all the fans that helped me, none did so in greater numbers than those of Cardiff City. Indeed, they provided me with one of the most touching tributes.

A few weeks after my surgery and in the early days of my treatment, I was invited by BBC Radio Wales to be their match summariser at Gillingham, who were playing Cardiff that day.

There were hundreds of Bluebirds fans behind the one goal and after a while they spotted me in the stands, armed with my microphone and headphones, doing the commentary. Almost as one they began chanting my name and encouraging me to 'do the Ayatollah' – a gesture for which the Cardiff fans have become famous.

I was so touched by that, at one stage I could hardly speak – which is far from ideal when you are being paid to talk on radio! They were singing my name as if I was still playing for them. They were fabulous.

Driving home, I can admit now, my eyes filled with tears as I thought about what had happened. I couldn't really take in why they were so good to me. After all, I'd been gone quite a few years from Ninian Park. Yet they still remembered me and again tried to lift me. Wonderful!

It was just another case of me being overwhelmed by the support and concern for the illness I had been fighting. I can honestly say to all those who contacted me, I have not thrown out one card, message or e-mail; I have them all.

When they were sent to me, I was lying in a caravan, which was home while my house was being built, sometimes so tired I couldn't move because of the treatment, but I was lifted by the goodwill of football fans far and wide.

It's a shame the newspapers and media don't make more of these sorts of gestures, to publicise what good football fans can do. I'll never throw away any of the messages. If I ever have to go through that sort of treatment again, I will definitely read through all the messages knowing they will help me. I am living proof of the power of football supporters as a force for good.

Chapter Five

Early Footballing Days

As a kid I had no thoughts of being a professional footballer. My brother Paul was always the better player, and had trials with Swansea, Cardiff, Shrewsbury and Hull. I remember him having one trial but then getting homesick, so he came home. I'm sure he could have made it.

I used to play in the morning and watch him in the afternoon because he was better than me. My football ability was summed up by the fact that I used to play in goal.

But the older I grew, the more interest there seemed to be in me as a player, because I was now playing in the outfield on the left side. I had two or three years in the Neath League before Pontardawe asked me to join them, and after a couple of months I joined Briton Ferry in the Welsh League.

That was a good standard, but still the thought of being a professional hadn't really crossed my mind. I was twenty-one, I had worked in the Forestry Commission and now I was a supervisor in a paint spraying section of a shelving systems factory. I used to enjoy my Friday nights out and would play football on Saturday.

Then one night we played at Aberystwyth, winning 3–2, and I scored twice. Coming off the field, the manager Alwyn Mainwaring told me there were three people to see me in the bar. I thought they would be journalists and said he should talk to them. He said they were representatives of clubs. One was from Wolves, one from Middlesbrough, the other from Swansea City. They were all interested in me and the next time I played, someone from Manchester City was watching me, as they also wanted me.

For some reason I chose Middlesbrough. I managed to get time off work and was invited to go up there for a couple of weeks, so they could have a look at me. Players like Gary Pallister, Tony Mowbray, Colin Cooper and Steven Pears were there.

Middlesbrough weren't in the top division at the time, but I used to love watching games at Ayresome Park, a ground they have now left for their new home at the Riverside Stadium. I even got to play up front in the reserves with Bernie Slaven, who was a legend at the club.

Their manager was Bruce Rioch, who was strict on players looking the part. He used to fine them for being scruffy, unshaven or wearing so-called 'designer' T-shirts which looked tatty. I was a long-haired kid at the time and it soon cost me.

One day, the players were in the dressing room when Bruce Rioch walked in and told us we were all fined £1. I remember Gary Pallister asking why. It was because of me, with my hair down to my shoulders. "He has to get his hair cut or he's going home," said Rioch. So after training I just got in my car and went back to Wales. Rioch rang me to see where I was, but that was it for me with Middlesbrough, which was a shame, really, because they had a good set-up there.

Soon I had a call to go to Manchester City, so again I had time off work for a trial there. I was told I had to report to their Maine Road ground at six o'clock for a reserve game. I walked from my hotel to the ground past an area which, admittedly, didn't look the best. There were even what looked to me like wire cages around the place.

When I arrived at the ground the doorman

said, "Where have you been?" I told him where I had come from and he looked shocked. He said, "You have just walked through Moss Side!" It was supposed to be a dodgy part of the city. I didn't have a clue.

I played one reserve game for Manchester City, up front alongside Imre Varadi at Maine Road. The manager Mel Machin wasn't there to see me and wanted me to return during the pre-season to see what my attitude was like and whether I would be fit enough for professional football.

But in the meantime, Swansea City manager Terry Yorath had been in touch and asked if I wanted to play for the Swans reserves against – of all clubs – Cardiff City, at the Vetch Field. What a game to be thrown into! Ceri Williams, Dudley Lewis and Ian Love all played for the Swans and little did I know how large the Swansea–Cardiff derby (admittedly at a more senior level) would feature in my life in the future.

Terry must have liked what he saw of me and soon I was combining training with working in the factory. Sometimes I would have to take time off to fit in the football and eventually Swansea City offered me a contract.

My job as a supervisor gave me decent

earnings and I was getting boot money from Briton Ferry, so I certainly didn't go into football for the cash on offer. It makes me laugh when I hear people talking about greedy footballers. I took a massive pay cut to join Swansea City.

I also had to change my lifestyle when I took the step into professional football, and I found that difficult. With plenty of money in my pocket, I'd been used to going out every Friday night. That had to stop when I turned pro.

I signed for the Swans in August 1988 and within the first two months I had a stress fracture of the leg, which slowed my progress. But I worked hard enough to earn a debut at Bristol City, marking Ralph Milne, who had already been sold to Manchester United. We lost 2–0 but I still have a video of the game.

Despite the result, I enjoyed everything about the occasion and the build-up, though some of it was entirely new for me, such as the pre-match meal. On Fridays, Tommy Hutchison, who was Terry's number two, would come into the dressing room and on a blackboard he would take down the orders for the pre-match meals.

When Tommy asked what I wanted, Ian Love told me to say "steak". So I said, "Steak and chips, please, Tom." At which point, the board duster came flying at me and Tommy told me I would have chicken. The rest of the lads just laughed.

When we got to the hotel, Terry Yorath sat beside me at the pre-match meal and checked I was okay. I told him I was nervous but fine. My chicken was brought to me but I didn't move. Terry said, "Don't you want to eat?" I said, "I'm waiting for the chips!" I didn't know any better, and got a mighty punch in the arm from Terry.

At half time, Terry asked me whether I was okay and whether I needed to ask him anything. I said, "Got any chocolate? I'm starving!" And I got beaten up for that as well.

As you will have gathered by now, I was quite naïve. I can't believe how gullible I was at Swansea as a young footballer starting on my professional career. In the dressing room the senior players soon picked up on that and I often had the mickey taken out of me.

The squad used to go to a place called Harpers in Swansea for our nights out but, because I was only twenty-two, Robbie James used to take me in – you had to be twenty-five. One day my team-mate Peter Bodak told me to ask the club secretary for my Harpers' pass. Being a bit dull, I did.

The next day Terry Yorath announced in training I would be receiving a presentation. He said, "Leggy, here's your Harpers' pass." I thought he was telling the truth. Instead, I had a verbal volley from him about being a professional footballer and watching my lifestyle. And he punched me – again!

But I'll never forget the chance Terry gave me, and I will always thank him for that. Not only did he take me on, he also toughened me up. I was a left winger who could run with the ball and get the odd goal. Terry and Tommy Hutchison made me much stronger, particularly mentally. They believed that if you were tough in the mind, you would be tough on the pitch. I've never forgotten that. They also hated losing and bred that into me.

Tommy spent hours on the training ground teaching me how to cross a ball without having to beat a man. Of course, he couldn't teach me how to cross with my right foot – that was just for standing on! But he did show me that I didn't have to beat a man to cross the ball. Again I will always be grateful.

Some of my career highlights came in a Swansea City shirt, and I was delighted when I was presented with a silver salver for playing one hundred and thirty-six consecutive league and cup games from March 1991 to the end of 1992–3 season. I was known for my fitness and my ability to get up and down the left wing whether at full back or further forward. And I was fortunate in avoiding injury.

I won the Welsh Cup with the Swans in 1989 and 1991 and I had the thrill of playing European football in the Cup Winners' Cup. We came across some big sides like the Greek club Panathinaikos, whom we played away from home in front of a crowd of more than 50,000.

We also played Monaco, who beat us 2–1 at the Vetch Field, our only goal coming from me. I was pleased to score against them because their team included future World Footballer of the Year George Weah, Emanuel Petit, Youri Djorkaeff and they were managed by Arsene Wenger. They were much too good for us in the second leg when we were thrashed 8–0. But just to cross swords with the likes of those players gave me a real buzz.

While I was at Swansea City, I also scored THE best goal of my career. I scored a few from outside the box but the best by far was against Stoke City with Bruce Grobelaar in goal. I still have the video – Russell Coughlin, who was a great passer of the ball, was on the right side of the pitch and when the ball came to me on the edge of the penalty area on the left, I volleyed it into the top corner. Grobelaar didn't have a chance, but as I celebrated he wagged his finger at me and said, "Never again!" He was right – I've never scored anything as good since, but I still wind him up about it when we meet on the golf course.

Chapter Six

Difficult Decisions

I had five happy years at the Swans, but when we lost to West Bromwich Albion in the Second Division play-off semi-final, I knew it was time to go. I think even the manager Frank Burrows realised I had stayed at the Vetch Field for long enough and had given good service to the club. Even after five years I wasn't on the best money and had stayed there for the football, definitely not the cash.

At the end of the 1993 season, I was aware that a number of clubs wanted me. I knew Wimbledon had been watching me. Frank would have liked me to go to Portsmouth, who offered me most money, and where the likeable Jim Smith was at the helm. I could have gone to Luton but didn't get a good feeling there. Ossie Ardiles was keen on me at West Bromwich Albion, but by the time I got back from holidays he had gone, so I ruled out that move.

Eventually I settled for Notts County whom I joined for a fee of £275,000. I negotiated my side of the deal myself, since all through my career I have never had an agent, which is rare these days. It's probably cost me a lot of money over the years, but I have always wanted to be in control of my own destiny. I felt Notts County wanted me more than any other club and so I took the plunge. Just as well, really, because it was in Nottingham that I met my wife – an unexpected bonus for the move to Meadow Lane.

Notts County were in what is known now as the Championship and in my first year there we just missed out on the play-offs, finishing seventh. But there were some terrific games with the division including Birmingham, West Bromwich Albion, Derby County, Stoke City, Middlesbrough, Sunderland and Nottingham Forest.

Despite relegation the next season, we also twice reached the Anglo–Italian Cup final at Wembley. We lost to Brescia in our first final in 1994, but beat Ascoli in the following year under manager Howard Kendall. I remember it well because one of the goals came from my long throw.

In the 1995–6 season, Notts County were

among the pace-setters for promotion in Division Two with me on the left wing and Paul Devlin on the right. But, much to our surprise, we were both left out of the side to play at Bournemouth one Tuesday night. Devlin went on as substitute, but I didn't play. The following day we were both told to report to the ground and when I saw the car of Birmingham manager Barry Fry in the car park, I was sure Devlin was on the move.

I suspected nothing and was told I had to speak to the local press about the game coming up on the Saturday. I didn't see Devlin, but once I had finished talking to the media, the Notts County chairman called me into his office and said, "I've just sold you to Birmingham." I told him I wasn't going anywhere because I was happy where I was, but Barry Fry was in the corner of the room and suddenly bellowed, "Sold to the Fat Bastard!"

That was the first time I had come across Barry and it was quite a first impression. He insisted, "I've signed the two of you, come down to St Andrews tomorrow and join a proper club." The Notts County chairman made it clear it would be in my best interests to make the move, though I told Barry I had to speak to Lucy about the switch before I signed anything.

But next day there I was at a new club and it was nothing like I was used to. At Notts County the training kit would be all laid out ready for me. At Birmingham there was nothing like that – so I did my first training session in Barry Fry's tracksuit bottoms, and an 'I love Lanzarote' T-shirt. I wore the same stuff for the press conference, too, posing for pictures holding a Birmingham City scarf.

For me, transferring to Birmingham was a big move, and it also started a friendship with Barry Fry which has lasted to this day. He's such a character. Some of his antics used to astonish me but he has been a really good friend.

I joined Birmingham in February 1996, though within months Barry Fry left the club and Trevor Francis, a former player who was a legend at St Andrews, became manager. He had played in Italy and because of that was really professional in his approach. He made certain everything about preparing for the game was correct, including our food. If Trevor had known I was actually eating burgers he would have killed me!

It was a time of great change with players

like Mike Newell, Barry Horne, Steve Bruce and Gary Ablett coming in. Again I was privileged to play alongside someone like Steve Bruce, who was an England international coming to the end of his career, but who still had great class.

I was at Birmingham for almost two years and during my time there I made my first appearance for Wales. The beginning of the end for me was when I started negotiating a new contract and, having rejected the terms, I was put in the reserves.

Trevor asked me if I wanted to go on loan to Ipswich, who were managed by George Burley. It was made clear to me I was going to Portman Road purely as cover for an injury to their player Bobby Petta, so there was no pressure. I could concentrate on playing without having to worry about my future.

But after a month, George said he wanted to sign me permanently. Before I went on loan to Ipswich, I had made a deal with Trevor Francis which meant I could leave Birmingham for a nominal sum. So imagine my surprise when George told me Ipswich had agreed a fee with Birmingham for me which was much more than was mentioned in my agreement with Trevor.

I was annoyed. I felt Trevor had reneged on a deal and I told him I was going nowhere unless I could have a cut of the transfer fee. In the end I didn't move and, on reflection, I was stupid. I should have gone to Ipswich. But I felt Trevor could be quite petty and he wanted his own way all the time. I had nothing else against him and have spoken to him since. But, at that time, if you fell out with him you knew it.

Soon afterwards Jason Bowen, my best mate, had left Birmingham for Reading. He was full of praise for a club who were building a new stadium and I joined him there in February 1988 – for £75,000.

Imagine my shock when, after just a handful of games for the Royals, the other players and I were having a day out at Cheltenham races when we all had phone calls saying the manager Terry Bullivant had been sacked.

Tommy Burns became manager – and brought a clutch of new players with him. Tommy divided the squad from almost the first minute he walked into the club. At the start I played a few games for him, but before long we fell out.

Tommy had pushed aside a few players,

including Jason, saying he didn't want the rest of the squad bothering with them. Jason just wasn't Tommy's cup of tea. Yet Jason was my best pal and I had no intention of spoiling our friendship.

In time, the disputes got worse. A group of us had nothing to do with the first team. They would train in the morning, and we would have a session with the reserve coach Alan Pardew in the afternoon. We were basically in internal exile. We were being paid by Reading, but not allowed to play a part in the club. Alan Pardew told us to dig in and keep our heads down – he was absolutely brilliant for us – but there was no way that state of affairs could continue.

Players and managers will always have disagreements, but Tommy Burns was the only boss with whom I fell out totally. He's the one manager I would have walked across the street to avoid because, though I have seen players who are not wanted at clubs, the way he treated us and some of the things he said to us were terrible. There was no need for it.

That said, after all I have been through in later years fighting cancer, I obviously felt for Tommy and his family when he died from the illness.

After less than a year and having made just a dozen league starts for Reading, I had to leave. Despite the good money, I just couldn't stay at the club without playing. Jason Bowen felt the same.

I had been on loan at Peterborough and could have gone there. But Jason and I met with Frank Burrows, my old boss at Swansea City, who was now manager at Cardiff City.

He wanted us both at Ninian Park, and I faced the most agonising football decision of my life.

Chapter Seven

Crossing the Great Divide

Everyone in football knows about the rivalry between Cardiff City and Swansea City. It's still one of the most notorious.

I had played in enough derbies for the Swans against the Bluebirds to know just how deep feelings ran between the supporters. I suppose the rivalry was worse when I played for the Swans.

But as I mulled over moving from Reading, I was concerned. Yes, I wanted to get away from a club where I was very unhappy and Frank Burrows was a manager I knew and respected from my days with Swansea City. But could I cross the great football divide and join Cardiff City?

I have played in plenty of derbies in different parts of the country during my time as a professional. I played for Birmingham against Midlands rivals. I played in the Nottingham derby, when you could certainly see the divide, but you could also see fans of Forest and County walking across the bridge together.

That didn't happen in the south Wales derby. I'd say the hatred between the fans – and that isn't a word I use lightly – was the most intense I had ever come across. Maybe because I was a local boy when I played for the Swans, I felt it intensely.

Even today very few players make the jump between Cardiff and Swansea. Alan Curtis and Robbie James played for both clubs and nailed it, because they were such good professionals. Jimmy Gilligan is also admired by both sets of fans, thanks to the service he gave to the two clubs.

But I was worried. I knew I would get stick from the Cardiff fans for being a former Swansea player and I also knew some sections of the Swans supporters wouldn't be happy. I wasn't sure I could turn it around and I didn't want to become another David Penney. He moved from Swansea directly to Cardiff and was hammered.

When I was at Swansea, there had been talk of me leaving for Cardiff. I think the then Bluebirds manager Eddie May wanted me. I remember seeing the headlines in the *South Wales Evening Post* about Cardiff's interest and thinking, I'm not sure I can go there. Frank Burrows, my Swansea boss, told me not to worry – I was going nowhere.

But now, a few years later, Frank was trying to persuade me and Jason Bowen, who had also started at the Swans, to go to Ninian Park – the home of the arch-rivals.

I think Frank was the only man who could have got me to make the move. I told him about my concerns for both myself and my family, but he kept telling me he was sure I could win over the Bluebirds fans.

I was also taking a cut of about half in my wages, so there were other considerations. But it was the situation of me being a former Swansea player joining Cardiff which really played on my mind.

In the end I decided to take the plunge and told Jason Bowen my decision, thinking he would probably come with me. I'll never forget his reply. He said, "You go first – I'll see how you get on!"

On the day I arrived at Ninian Park I was met by a few players I already knew, like Dai Thomas, Rob Earnshaw, Lee Phillips and Scott Young. They all made a fuss of me. Scott Young called me a 'Jack'.

I was on the bench for my first game in Cardiff colours against Mansfield, at Ninian Park. When they announced my name before the match there were boos from some of the home fans. During the game, I went to warm up in front of Ninian's famous Grange End and some of the Cardiff supporters spat at me. After the match Jason Bowen rang me to see how it had gone. I was honest with him. "They're hammering me."

He said, "Well, I'm not coming yet!"

We had similar chats for quite a while. I scored my first goal for Cardiff at Plymouth. I knew the fans of the two clubs didn't get on, so I thought that goal would turn the Bluebirds supporters in my favour. As soon as I scored I went to celebrate in front of the away fans section at Home Park. But they hurled abuse and threw things at me. I just couldn't win.

I got back on the team bus for the trip home and I had calls from my wife and Jason Bowen. Lucy said I must be delighted, so was surprised when I told her I still had flak from the Cardiff fans. Jason said he'd probably be down to join me at the club next week. I said, "Don't bother – they're still spitting at me!"

I also scored at Rochdale and the same

thing happened. I was being jeered by both sets of fans in any game I played!

Abusive mail also came my way, including some death threats. I can remember Winston Faber opening a letter of mine and slashing the top of his finger because there was a razor blade inside the envelope. I was beginning to wonder whether I would ever get the fans on my side.

Then it all changed for me in a Football Association of Wales Premier Cup derby against Swansea City, at Ninian Park. Jimmy Goodfellow was Cardiff's physiotherapist and when we were talking about the criticism I was getting from the fans he said, "You know what you have to do, don't you?"

I said, "Yes, score a goal."

He said, "No. You have to clatter somebody."

Luckily for me, I caught a Swans player in the first three or four minutes of the game. I think the unfortunate fall guy was Stuart Roberts, but frankly, it could have been any of the players.

Jimmy Goodfellow was absolutely correct. From that moment the Cardiff supporters hardly stopped chanting my name during the match and when I went home I said to Lucy, "I think I've done it."

Frank Burrows always said that if any player couldn't handle criticism, he shouldn't play the game. He instilled into me that if I tried for the shirt and the fans, they would accept even bad performances. What supporters found unacceptable was any player not trying.

Jason Bowen soon followed me to Ninian Park and he also won them over, though he could always do more with the ball than I could. He had no problems ability-wise. I didn't have anywhere near his talent so I had to work hard for all my rewards.

These days there seem to be fewer lads staying with their local club and featuring in the derby match. In the old days there were the likes of Jason Perry, Damon Searle, Scott Young and Nathan Blake playing for Cardiff. All were boys from the south Wales area. The Swans had Steve Jenkins, Chris Coleman, Andy Melville, Jason Bowen and me. To me, the derby meant more and was fiercer then because of the local boys, living in the area, alongside the fans who couldn't stomach losing to their arch rivals.

If I was in the professional game now, I'd still think twice about moving between Cardiff and Swansea, though I think it's easier going from Ninian Park to the Liberty Stadium, which is now the Swans' home. Few players still make the switch directly and the fear of consequences could help explain why the numbers are so low.

But I was so glad I plucked up the courage to move to Cardiff City, because I went on to have an unforgettable time there.

Chapter Eight

Never a Dull Moment

My time at Cardiff City was eventful to say the least.

We were promoted from Division Three in my first season, relegated the next, then promoted once more the following campaign. After that there were two promotion play-offs – the final one ending with Cardiff promoted to the Championship at the Millennium Stadium.

Throw in five different managers and the arrival of the colourful chairman Sam Hammam, and you can see why there was never a dull moment.

I don't think you could get a more varied bunch of managers. Frank Burrows had total respect from everyone and was brilliant at keeping you on your toes. Billy Ayre was one of the toughest men I ever met and wanted to win on and off the pitch. Bobby Gould was a real character, though he didn't have much of a chance at Cardiff and went 'upstairs' to a

Director of Football role. Alan Cork was a players' bloke. And Lenny Lawrence was thoughtful in everything he did.

As for Sam Hammam, well, no one who knows him will be surprised to learn that most of the outrageous stories you hear about him are true. At Cardiff he transformed the whole place.

I'll never forget the day he walked in. We were at the training ground and he paid someone to let down the tyres of the players' cars. I think the rate was £5 a tyre. When we came off the pitch, we immediately blamed the apprentices, while Sam was there trying to sell us a pump – for a tenner!

Alan Cork was the manager and said we had to teach Sam a lesson and take revenge for what he had done. The squad used to eat in a room upstairs, so I gathered together a bin load of canteen waste including stinking water, slops of food and cigarette ash, and got 'Corky' to lure Sam for a chat which would take place below the balcony. Sam walked into the trap and I poured the entire contents of the bin over his head. I can remember him saying, "Welcome to World War Three!"

The 'war' went on for three or four weeks. He took the buttons off my shirts and cut my socks in half. I took the bolts off his windscreen wipers when it was raining and stuffed a banana into the exhaust of his car. We eventually called a truce.

I think I was a bit of a golden boy for Sam, who would take me to his famous meetings with the Cardiff fans. He was unpredictable, and would call you in if you were on low money and just give you a pay rise without you having to ask.

Having lived in the area, I knew how big the support could be for Cardiff City. Sam transformed the scene and got the fans interested and talking about the club again. A few years before I arrived at Cardiff City, the businessman Rick Wright had built up the club only to vanish, and the whole place went on the slide. Sam had his critics, but he roused the club again when he walked through the door.

I was frequently written off as a player at Ninian Park, but I kept seeing off contenders for my place and played a part in three Cardiff promotions. Easily the most memorable was in 2003 when the Bluebirds appeared in the Division Two play-off final against Queens Park Rangers, at the Millennium Stadium. For me it was my top day in sport, with more than

66,000 there. It was a day which will live with me for ever.

I was pinching myself that it was happening to me at the age of thirty-six. Cardiff had been trying to get rid of me for a while and I was now playing in front of a full house. Andy Campbell scored the goal which will always have a special part in the club's history, to give us a 1–0 win, and Cardiff were into the second tier of English football for the first time for eighteen years. I had been proud to play for Wales, but this day was unbelievable.

Yet after the elation came the biggest disappointment of my career – I was out of the club. Before the play-off final, the manager Lenny Lawrence had told me I would get another year's deal. My wife was delighted because we were building a house in the Bridgend area at the time. After the play-off win, Lenny told me to go away and enjoy my holidays before the start of the next pre-season.

But out of the blue, I had a phone call from Lenny calling me in for a meeting. There I was told I could have a new contract, but would have to take a 70 per cent pay cut. I can remember an article in the local paper with

Sam Hammam asking me not to go and saying it would be like 'Pele leaving Santos'. I wondered what Pele would have thought of such a pay cut.

Lucy, who initially hadn't been keen on south Wales, was as disappointed as I was. We had moved into a new house and lived there for only five weeks. But we had to leave.

The Cardiff fans' reaction to my departure was unbelievable because they knew I wanted to stay. Their backing was an indication of what was to come when I fought my second cancer battle.

Sam and I gave each other some stick in the press for a while, but I made it up with him the following year when I travelled back from playing at Blackpool for a Cardiff City Supporters Club event. Sam was there. I tapped him on the shoulder and he said, "I still love you, Leggy baby," and we have spoken ever since. Life's too short to hold grudges.

As one door shut, another opened and I was lucky, I had people interested in me when I left Cardiff.

I decided on Peterborough, because I'd got on well with Barry Fry both at Birmingham and in a loan spell with Posh, as Peterborough is known. Also he was prepared to offer me a player–coach role.

I went on to play more than seventy League games for Peterborough, my League-playing career cut short by my second tumour in April 2005.

But the treatment didn't end my connection with Peterborough. When I was recovering, Barry asked me to train there, and I also did scouting reports and some coaching sessions.

The club was skint and Barry was putting everything into it. I think some of the fans thought he was ripping them off, but financially Barry was risking everything on a club he loved.

During that time, Ron Atkinson brought the cameras into the club to film for a programme, *Big Ron Manager.* That was certainly different because the cameras were allowed total access.

Later, I joined Llanelli in the Welsh Premier League, to keep myself fit as much as anything, which the doctor thought would be a good idea in the battle with my illness.

Then I left Llanelli for a while, to move closer to my Nottingham home and play for Hucknall Town. And while I was there, the manager Kevin Wilson got the sack and the chairman asked me to take on the job.

So I walked into my first manager's post without really thinking about it. I was still playing, taking training, scouting, watching other games and had no assistant. I was on my own. My term lasted six games into the next season before I resigned. I don't regret taking the job and one day I would like another crack at management. But I'll go into it with my eyes open.

Chapter Nine

Playing for Wales

I'm proud to be Welsh and there's no bigger honour than playing for your country. I cherished every moment I was involved with Wales.

I got the call-up when I was at Birmingham and was surprised. I don't suppose I should have been because my manager at Notts County, Colin Murphy, always reckoned I had a chance of a cap when I was playing for them.

"Worse players than you have played for Wales, Leggy. You should be in the squad," Colin used to say, in his own distinctive style. Even though Colin kept on about it all the time I thought he was winding me up. I used to chuckle to myself, never thinking it was going to happen, even though I was hitting form and scoring goals.

But having moved to Birmingham, I got the call. Strange really, because I thought I was playing in a better team at Notts County.

Perhaps it happened because I was at a bigger club, but I was still delighted.

I had to pinch myself on Wales duty because I was in squads with Ryan Giggs, Neville Southall, Gary Speed, Barry Horne and Mark Hughes. Sparky had been at Barcelona and just to be on the same training ground as him was fantastic. I remember being with Robbie Savage, who was at Crewe at the time. We would just sit there in the hotel and be as quiet as we could, though for Robbie that wasn't easy.

The experience was amazing, though my debut was anything but. It was away to Switzerland in Lugano in April 1996 and it lasted precisely twenty-five minutes. It was 0–0 when I went down the wing, and I was just going to cross the ball when I damaged my ankle ligaments. I had to go off and we lost 2–0. What a Wales bow!

What really surprised me was something which happened on the journey home. One of the committee men came up to me and said what a good trip it had been. I asked him why. He said they had been well looked after by the Swiss. I couldn't believe what I was hearing. My debut had lasted less than half the game, I'd hurt my ankle and was facing six weeks on the sidelines with the injury. But the committee men had been well treated, so it was a good trip!

I found just being involved in the squad a pleasure. I loved meeting up with all the lads, even though I didn't play that often. In training I'd be surrounded by players who were my heroes – it couldn't get any better.

I was never one to look out for the squad every time it was announced. But I enjoyed every time I got the call – and that was far more often than the six occasions I actually represented my country. I was like many Welsh players even today – I used to go to squad training sessions knowing I wouldn't be in the first eleven.

I was always honest with myself as a player. I knew I wasn't at the top of the tree. I was never going to be a Giggs or a Speed. I knew I was never going to be as good as Mark Hughes. They were top-flight players and I was not. I accepted that but was chuffed every time I pulled on a Welsh shirt.

And the great thing was, even Wales's very best players accepted players like me. I was always made to feel welcome and they would never put people like me down.

Some of our players were superstars. To my mind I played with the best keeper in the world at the time – Neville Southall. Not many could say that. I also played with the best left-winger in the world – Ryan Giggs.

I would have loved to have played for my country in the finals of a major championship, but players like Kevin Ratcliffe, Mark Hughes, Ryan Giggs and Neville Southall really deserved it. It was their proper stage, and I feel desperately sorry for those players who didn't get to play for Wales in the major championship their talent deserved.

For all the stars we had, we were still all one squad. It was never a case of "I'm a superstar – you're a muppet."

Having said that, when I first joined the squad I was very nervous. We used to get together in Newport, and I remember one morning we were having a work-out when Dean Saunders asked me if I wanted to play golf later.

Being a keen golfer I immediately said 'yes'. But the manager Bobby Gould had told the squad there was no golf allowed that day, so I couldn't help wondering whether they were setting me up.

When I got back to the hotel, I tiptoed

down the stairs to check the others were there at the appointed time. Dean Saunders and John Hartson were waiting for me – and they had their golf clubs. I raced back upstairs to get my own.

But when I got down to meet the others Bobby Gould had spotted us. "I thought I told you no golf," he said. Dean Saunders told him all the buggies had been booked. Bobby relented. "Just nine holes then."

I must admit I got on well with Bobby Gould, though plenty of players did not. I was a substitute in Italy when he resigned after a 4–0 defeat. It was the first time I'd been present when a manager quit.

The instructions beforehand were to keep things tight for the first twenty minutes or so. But Christian Vieri scored for Italy after about six minutes and by half time we were 3–0 down. At the interval there was a bit of a row, I think over Dean Saunders being replaced by John Hartson and I'm certain Bobby said he was going to resign. At the end of the game he did just that.

I have to say there were some happy faces amongst the Welsh squad, who were glad to see him go. Bobby was always fine with me and, in fact, in later years he seemed to follow me around because I was with him at Cardiff and Peterborough.

Neville Southall and Mark Hughes took over the Welsh managerial reins when Bobby packed it in because we had a game against Denmark at Anfield, Liverpool a few days later. I didn't see Bobby for quite some time after the trip to Italy.

As I said earlier, I played just the six times for Wales, though the last one was unexpected. I hadn't been involved for nearly two years when Mark Hughes called me up for a World Cup qualifier in Armenia in 2001.

I had never felt upset about being overlooked and had always taken squad announcements with a pinch of salt. But to be recalled at the age of thirty-two by Sparky, for whom everyone in the game has so much respect, was something special.

It certainly didn't turn out to be my best game for Wales. I am honest enough to admit I made a mistake leading up to their first goal and we ended up drawing 2–2.

But just to be involved again was brilliant for me, and was another occasion I will recall with pride because I was playing for my country. Pulling on the red shirt for Wales is another reason why my football career has been so enjoyable.

Chapter Ten

My World Record Throw-in

Before my illness there's no doubt what I was best known for – my long throw.

It's unusual for a footballer who is not a goalkeeper to be famous for the use of his hands, but it is absolutely true in my case. Wherever I go people invariably ask me about my long throw.

To be honest, I don't know how or why I can throw the ball so far. When I was a kid of thirteen or fourteen someone mentioned I seemed to be able to throw the ball quite a way at throw-ins, but no big deal was made of it.

People started to talk about it more when I played for Briton Ferry in the Welsh League. I remember someone saying, "My God ... look how far you can throw that ball!"

I used to wonder what the fuss was all about. As far as I was concerned I just used to throw the ball into the box. I thought everyone could do it.

When I signed for Swansea City, Terry Yorath encouraged me to use my throw. In fact, every now and then he used to get one of the coaches, Ronnie Walton, to get me to throw a really heavy medicine ball in training for practice.

When we played Greek side Panathinaikos in a European game, we used it to great effect and the more we did that at Swansea, the more word seemed to get around about it. At one time, I know, Wimbledon were watching me and it was easy to see why they might want me. With the combination of my throw and their long ball tactics, I was a pretty obvious target.

Another Swansea manager, Frank Burrows, used to wind me up about it and on one hot sunny day he threatened me with extra training in the afternoon if I couldn't clear half the length of the pitch with a throw-in. I put in a big effort and did it!

Shoot magazine also did a feature on me and pictured the stages of my throw. When I looked at their spread, I was amazed just where my arms went as I leaned back to take the throw. My arms were almost down to my backside! (I still use the throws when I play, but old age has started to catch up with me and I can't get my arms that far back now.)

Interest really picked up when I got a place in the *Guinness Book of World Records*. I had to go to Wembley where they held a competition before an England game against Brazil. It was a wet night and we had to step over television cables when we took the throw.

I actually threw it 44.6 metres. It was a record beaten a few years later by Dave Challinor, who was known as "Exocet" because of his long throws. But I was chuffed to set a world record.

Engineering experts at Cardiff University could hardly believe I was able to throw the ball so far. Unlike Dave Challinor, who is well over six feet tall, I am just 5'8", and it wasn't as if I was lifting weights in my spare time to increase my muscular strength.

The scientists decided to use me as a guinea pig for some experiments. So I went for tests in which my chest and arms were wired as I threw the ball. Unfortunately, the experiments took place indoors so I couldn't throw it too hard or too high. And when I went to throw the ball the wires just flew off, so I don't think they learned a great deal.

I put my ability down to technique; the main effect it used to have on me was sore abdominal muscles after matches. I had no problems with my back – I just felt like I had done a thousand press-ups.

But once my throw was known about there was no stopping managers asking me to use it, both to get the team up-field and out of defence as well as to throw the ball into the opposition's penalty box. Sometimes I would do an endless amount of running in games, just to switch to the opposite wing to take a throw.

And it could get boring. I remember one game when Peterborough played Tranmere, who had Dave Challinor in their ranks and all it seemed to be was a series of long throws from him or me.

The long throw is really nothing new, but you would hardly know that given the amount of publicity Rory Delap had for his throws when Stoke City got into the Premier League. That made me laugh, because Premier League defences just weren't used to it. Rory's been doing that in the lower leagues for years.

I must admit I used to get a bit peeved at people saying all I could do was throw the ball. I used to score my fair share of goals, made a few goals with my crosses and I would say there was a lot more to my game than a long throw.

I used to think it was an added bonus.

The manager who got most out of my throws was Alan Cork, at Cardiff City. But at Birmingham I played with big Kevin Francis, and at Notts County there was Devon White – they were both tall players and both loved my throws. On my Birmingham debut Kevin Francis told me to throw the ball at the goalkeeper. I did as he said, and he buried their keeper into the back of the net, and we won the game because the poor bloke was scared to come off his line for the rest of the game!

Of course, if you know your football, you'll also know you can't score direct from a throw-in. But I reckon I've actually scored three times from my throws.

In 1995 I played in the Anglo–Italian Cup final for Notts County against Ascoli, at Wembley. Early in the game I took a long throw, the keeper came for it and missed it, and the referee thought our striker Tony Agana had touched it and the goal was given. It actually went down as an own goal, but I'm convinced nobody actually touched it. And we won the game.

I also 'scored' for Llanelli in a European match when a goalkeeper came for the throw. The referee thought the ball had touched his gloves and so that goal was awarded too. And in a Welsh Premier League game for Llanelli, the opposing goalkeeper touched the ball with his gloves and that goal was rightly given.

So to my mind I've scored three times and haven't been given any of the goals. I believe there should be a change in the law. After all, a goalkeeper can score a goal, a player can score direct from a corner, a player can score direct from a free kick. It's time to allow goals direct from a throw-in!

Even without those 'goals', my long throws have earned me a world record and plenty of publicity. It's one of those things that I'm stuck with. Strange to say I'm a footballer who is most famous for throwing the ball. Or at least that's how it was until I got cancer ...

Chapter Eleven

Nagging Fears

"It'll kill you one day." Those blunt words came from the specialist Patrick Bradley.

It was stark but I appreciated his honesty. There was no point in him lying. I wouldn't have wanted him to, because he was straight with me from the first day I met him.

Every six months, I go to hospital to check the cancer hasn't returned. A few months after I'd finished the treatment I was sent for a full body scan. The results were fine and Patrick, being such a positive person, told me, "Go and enjoy your life."

When I go back to see him now he has to put his fingers almost down my throat to check there's no problem in the area where the two tumours appeared. It's uncomfortable and must look terrible, but I'm used to it. I don't need scans now, though Lucy sometimes feels I should have a second opinion. But as far as I am concerned Patrick is the top man and I have full trust in him.

There are still certain parts of the neck which are numb and you can still see the scar. But I feel well, I am well and I've been coaching and playing for Llanelli in the Welsh Premier League.

Of course, the fear of the cancer returning is always there. I can't say I think about it every day, and sometimes I might go a week or two without giving it a thought. But I don't consider myself out of the woods yet – and the threat of it returning is always there in the background.

Very occasionally I wonder if I can feel a lump, particularly as the feeling is starting to come back into my neck. I may be shaving and think something is sore because the feeling has returned. And the minute I feel some pain, particularly in the neck area, then I do wonder about the cancer. But that is just human nature.

Patrick Bradley told me not to look for cancer, instead just enjoy my life, though he added, "It'll kill you one day ... but then we've all got to die of something."

In other words, the chances are that the

cancer will return at some time. It could be two years, could be five years, it could be ten years or longer. I'm not sitting around worrying about it. I could die of a heart attack, get knocked over crossing the road or even die of old age!

If I get to five years in the clear I will feel I have a good chance of another twenty or thirty years free of it. That's the way I look at it.

Although I had to quit professional football, I remain in good shape because I am playing the game part-time, and I know Patrick thought my overall fitness had helped get me through all my treatment.

As I've said, I've never had a problem with putting on weight through eating too much, and I'll never forget the time a while after my cancer treatment I went to do some summarising at a game for BBC Radio Wales.

It was a boring goalless draw between Northampton and Wrexham. But for me it was a special day – I had the first burger since my treatment!

I know Geoffrey Boycott has changed his lifestyle and the things he eats since he suffered from cancer in a similar place to me. I have not. My wife tries to make sure I eat properly at home but when I'm not there she knows exactly what I am eating, and it usually involves a burger. I can't change.

Another thing that has not changed is the fear of that word 'cancer'. Even when people ask how I am they don't mention it. They might call it the 'Big C' but they often don't use the actual word. They are frightened of it. They should not be – because cancer is no longer a death sentence in this world, providing it is caught early enough.

Though writing this book has provided a wonderful opportunity for me to thank those who supported me in my cancer fight, there is a much more important message which I believe is vital to get across.

If anyone feels a lump on their body or a part of their skin changes colour for no reason then please, please, go to the doctor and get it checked out. I promise you, the doctor will not think you are wasting his or her time.

A message which came across to me loud and clear from the medical people who were treating me is that if the cancer is caught early enough, they have a much better chance of dealing with it.

And, I must emphasise, I don't feel like a

dead man walking. Caught early, cancer can be beaten. Not so long ago a cartilage or ligament problem often spelt the end of a footballer's career – now they are back in action a few weeks later with no more than keyhole surgery. So has the treatment of cancer improved.

As I've said earlier, I was very matter-of-fact about my first tumour. I didn't realise the seriousness of it. Don't make the same mistake as me. I was just very lucky.

In this book I've had a chance to reflect about the time I have spent fighting a problem which may come back to kill me one day.

Thinking back, I'm struck by the amount of work and preparation which goes into getting someone like me ready for treatment which can be life-saving, or at least can prolong life and make the quality of life better. The doctors and nurses involved are dedicated perfectionists. We should all be grateful for the work they do.

If the cancer does return, at least I know what I might have to go through again. It would worry me – but it wouldn't stop me fighting. Because in the battle against something like this, I'm not just fighting for myself. There are other people involved – Lucy, my daughter Alicia, my mum and the rest of my family and friends. I got through twenty-eight radiotherapy treatments, even though it was an intense struggle, because I was thinking about my wife and my daughter.

I didn't want them to see me dying. My daughter has ponies, and I want to see her enjoying her life. I want to see her leaving school and going to college. I want to see her grow up. I want to take my daughter down the aisle. There's still so much I want to do.

I also want to continue enjoying life with Lucy. We've been together for more than fifteen years and sometimes I wonder why, because she's had so much to put up with. I've got to give her a lot of credit and though I have probably never told her this – she has been my rock. She gave me the life I have at the moment.

On a recent visit to see Patrick Bradley, he pulled out a card from his desk from Geoffrey Boycott. It was a picture of a pair of fingers giving a 'V' sign. Boycott had signed it: "I'm still here after five years." What a great attitude.

Should my cancer flare again, it will be harder knowing the pain that might follow. I certainly wouldn't look forward to wearing that damned mask again, though I'm told they have changed a lot since I had to wear mine.

But more and more people are beating this ailment, and the treatment is getting better as technology and medicine improve. Fighting cancer now is easier rather than harder. I would be pretty confident.

Yes, the cancer might kill me one day, but I've got a different outlook on life now. Through adversity I've seen so much that is good, particularly with all the help and support I have had from my family, friends and the football world.

I am still enjoying being involved in football, whether it be playing or coaching. I am also enjoying my golf and fishing. I'm even still tucking into burgers.

As far as I'm concerned I'm legging it away from the Big C – and I'm very definitely 'Alive and Kicking.'

Inside Out

Real life stories from behind bars

Brought together by their crimes, the prisoners at Parc Prison, Bridgend, share their stories of life on the other side of the security walls.

Whether they are tough criminals or teenagers in trouble for the first time, they all have one thing in common – they had a life outside.

The prisoners have put into words what it's really like doing time at Parc Prison, how they got there and their hopes for the future.

These stories of their lives before crime will surprise and move you, make you laugh and cry in equal measures!

Royalties from this book will go to Parc Prison's arts and educational fund to support creative workshops for prisoners.

www.accentpress.co.uk

Black-Eyed Devils

Catrin Collier

One look was enough. Amy Watkins and Tom Kelly were in love. But that one look condemned them both.

'Look at Amy again and you'll return to Ireland in a box.' Amy's father is out to kill Tom.

All Tom wants is Amy and a wage that will keep them. But Tonypandy in 1911 is a dangerous place for Irish workers like Tom, who have been brought in to replace the striking miners. The miners drag them from their beds and hang them from lamp posts as a warning to those who would take their jobs.

Frightened for Amy, Tom fights to deny his heart, while Amy dreams of a future with the man she loves. But in a world of hatred, anger and violence, her dream seems impossible until a man they believed to be their enemy offers to help. But, can they trust him with their lives?

www.accentpress.co.uk

In At The Deep End: From Barry To Beijing

David Davies

As he was carried off on a stretcher at the Olympics in Beijing, Welsh swimmer David Davies was celebrating his success. He'd won a silver medal in one of the toughest races in the Olympics.

He also won a place in British swimming history as the first male swimmer to win medals at two consecutive Olympic Games in over thirty years.

In At The Deep End: From Barry To Beijing is David's own story of the highs and lows of his career. How a lanky schoolboy from Barry made the swimming world sit up and take notice. From his first success at the Commonwealth Games at the age of 17, he has gone on to win medals at every major championship. And he's still only 24.

www.accentpress.co.uk

Quick Reads

Books in the Quick Reads Series

www.quickreads.org.uk.